5 yoga poses to treat irregular periods

Yoga for a Healthy Menstrual Cycle

BY

ALVIA ASPEN

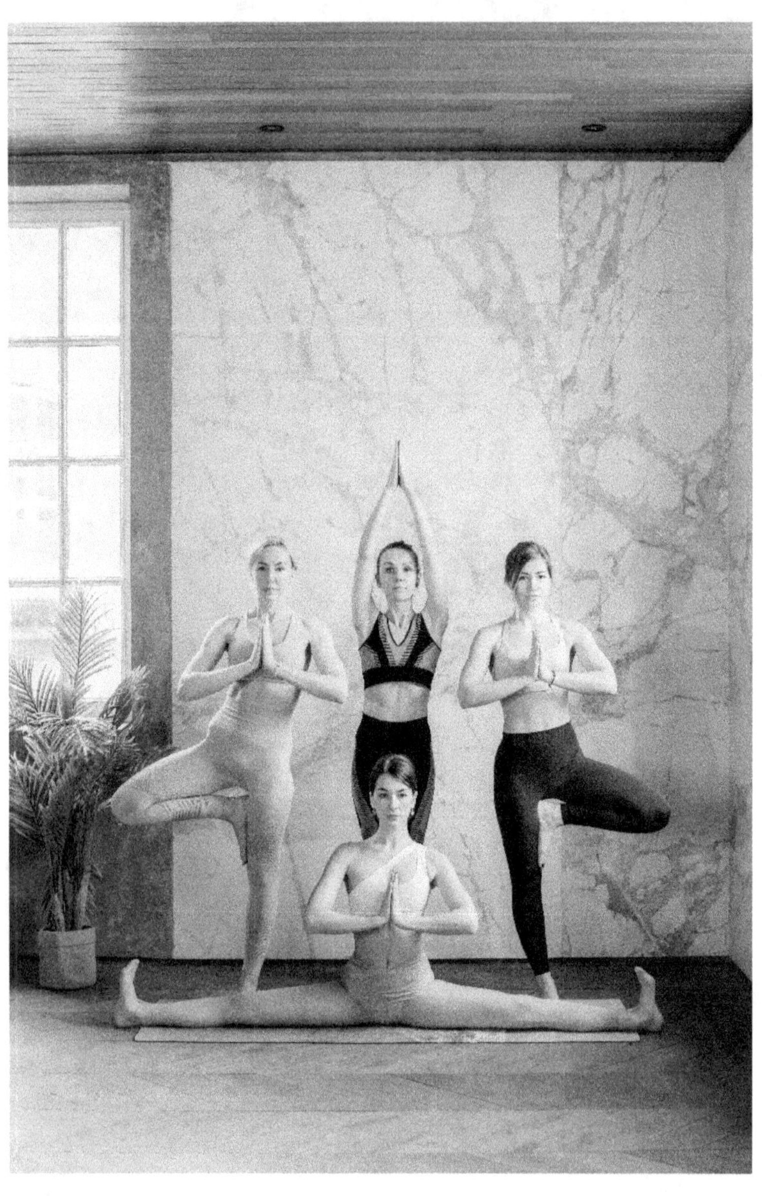

TABLE OF CONTENT

PART 1

The Menstrual Cycle

The menstrual cycle is a natural process that happens in women's bodies every month. It is a complex process that involves the interaction of hormones, the ovaries, and the uterus.

The menstrual cycle has four phases:

- The follicular phase: This is the phase when the egg matures in the ovary

- The ovulation phase: This is the phase when the egg is released from the ovary.

- The luteal phase: This is the phase when the egg travels through the fallopian tube to the uterus.

- The menstrual phase: This is the phase when the lining of the uterus is shed.

PART 2

5 Yoga Poses for a Healthy Menstrual Cycle

There are many yoga poses that can be beneficial for menstrual health. Some of the most beneficial poses include:

- Cat-cow pose

- Pigeon pose

- Spinal twist

- Corpse pose

- Yoga Nidra

PART 3

BREATHING Techniques for a Healthy Menstrual Cycle

Breathing techniques can also be beneficial for menstrual health. Some of the most beneficial breathing techniques include:

- Ujjain breath: This is a deep, calming breath that can help to reduce stress and anxiety.

- Kapalabhati breath: This is a cleansing breath that can help to improve circulation and oxygen levels.

- Anulom Vilom breath: This is a balancing breath that can help to promote relaxation and focus.

PART 4

Meditation for a Healthy Menstrual Cycle

Meditation can also be beneficial for menstrual health. Meditation can help to reduce stress, improve mood, and increase self-awareness.

There are many different types of meditation, so you can find one that works best for you. Some popular types of meditation for menstrual health include:

- Mindfulness meditation: This involves focusing on the present moment without judgment.

- Transcendental meditation: This involves repeating a mantra silently to oneself.

- Guided meditation: This involves listening to a guided meditation recording.

FINAL PART

Tips for Practicing Yoga for Menstrual Health

Here are some tips for practicing yoga for menstrual health:

• Practice regularly. The more you practice, the more benefits you will experience.

• Listen to your body. If a pose is too challenging, modify it or come out of it.

• Be patient. It takes time for the body to adjust to yoga. Don't expect to see results overnight.

Here are some additional tips for practicing yoga during your period:

• Avoid strenuous poses.

• Listen to your body and rest if you need to.

• Drink plenty of fluids.

• Avoid caffeine and alcohol

• Conclusion

BENEFITS AND IMPORTANCE OF YOGA

WHAT IS YOGA?

Yoga is a mind-body practice with a 5,000- time history in ancient Indian gospel. Colorful styles of yoga combine physical postures, breathing exercises, and contemplation or relaxation.

The word" yoga" comes from the Sanskrit word yuj, which means to unite or servitude. In yoga practice, the thing is to unite the mind, body, and spirit. This is done through a variety of ways, including physical postures, breathing exercises, and contemplation.

BENEFITS OF YOGA

Yoga has been displayed to have many advantages for feminine cycle wellbeing. A portion of the advantages of yoga for the feminine cycle include:

Diminished torment and squeezing: Yoga can assist with diminishing agony and squeezing by expanding dissemination and adaptability in the pelvic region.

Further developed flow: By encouraging the circulation of blood throughout the body, yoga can help improve circulation. This can assist with diminishing agony and squeezing, and work on generally speaking well-being.

Diminished pressure and uneasiness: Yoga can assist with decreasing pressure and uneasiness by advancing unwinding and care. This can be useful for ladies who experience feminine issues or different side effects that are exacerbated by pressure.

Controlled chemicals: Yoga can assist with directing chemicals by adjusting the body's regular rhythms. This can assist with further developing feminine cycle routineness and diminish side effects like PMS.

Further developed rest: Yoga can assist with further developing rest by advancing unwinding and lessening pressure. This can be useful for ladies who experience trouble resting during their feminine cycle.

Heightened levels of energy: Yoga can assist with expanding energy levels by further developing dissemination and adaptability. This can be useful for ladies who feel drained or exhausted during their feminine cycle.

Advanced unwinding: Yoga can assist with advancing unwinding by quieting the psyche and body. This can be useful for ladies who experience feminine issues or different side effects that are exacerbated by pressure.

IMPORTANCE OF YOGA

Yoga is a brain body practice that joins actual stances, breathing activities, and contemplation or unwinding.

Yoga has been displayed to have various advantages for physical and emotional wellness, etc.

Yoga is a protected and viable practice for individuals of any age and wellness levels. It tends to be finished at home or in a yoga studio. In the event that you are new to yoga, it is vital to begin gradually and continuously increment the force of your training.

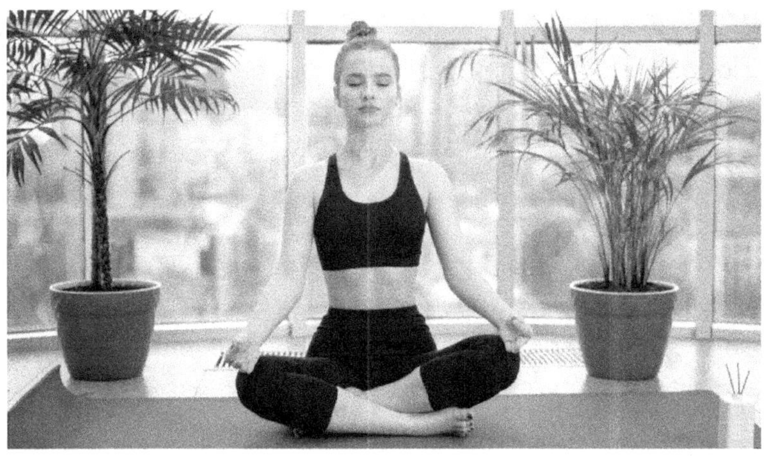

HOW TO APPROACH 30 DAYS CHALLENGE TO GET MAXIMAL RESULTS?

Notwithstanding, I can offer some broad way-of-life tips that might advance hormonal equilibrium and by and large prosperity:

Counsel a Medical services Supplier: Before endeavoring any test, talk with a gynecologist or medical services supplier to grasp the hidden reason for your unpredictable periods and to guarantee it's protected to seek after way of life changes.

Adjusted Diet: Center around an even eating routine wealthy in natural products, vegetables, entire grains, lean proteins, and sound fats. Keep away from unreasonable sugar, refined carbs, and handled food sources.

Normal Activity: Participate in customary active work, like strolling, running, cycling, or yoga. Exercise can assist with overseeing weight, lessen pressure, and back by and large hormonal equilibrium.

Stress The board: Persistent pressure can influence chemical levels and periods. Practice pressure-decrease strategies like contemplation, profound breathing activities, care, or side interests you appreciate.

Satisfactory Rest: Guarantee you are getting sufficient quality rest every evening. Hold back nothing long stretches of rest to help hormonal guidelines and by and large wellbeing.

Limit Caffeine and Liquor: High caffeine and liquor admission can affect chemical equilibrium. Balance is vital, or think about removing them however long the test might last.

Remain Hydrated: Drink a lot of water over the day to remain hydrated.

Abstain from Smoking: If you smoke, consider stopping, as smoking can upset the hormonal equilibrium and worsen feminine anomalies.

Track Your Cycle: Track your feminine cycle to screen any progressions or enhancements during the 30-day challenge.

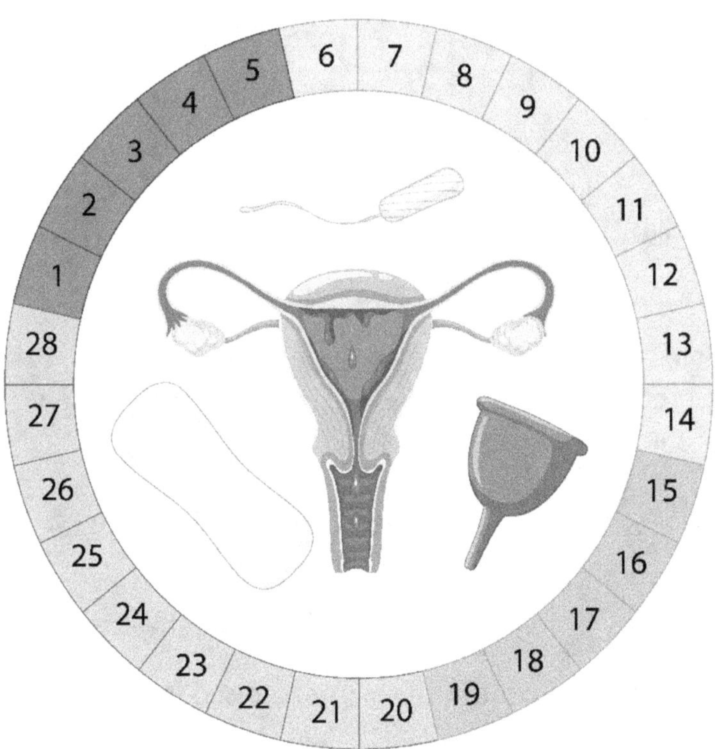

Homegrown Enhancements: A few homegrown supplements, such as chaste berry (Vitex), have been generally used to help chemical equilibrium. Notwithstanding, talk with your medical services supplier before attempting any enhancements.

In any case, I can offer a general eating regimen graph that advances, by and large, well-being and may uphold hormonal equilibrium. Recall that singular dietary necessities shift, so this diagram may not suit everybody:

Week 1:

Breakfast: Greek yogurt with berries and a sprinkle of nuts or seeds.

Early in the day bite: A piece of natural product (e.g., apple, pear, or berries).

Lunch: Barbecued chicken or tofu salad with blended greens, cucumber, tomatoes, and a light vinaigrette dressing.

Evening Bite: Carrot sticks with hummus.

Dinner: Heated salmon or a veggie pan sear with earthy-colored rice.

Week 2:

Breakfast: Spinach and mushroom omelet with entire grain toast.

Early in the day bite: A small bunch of almonds or pecans.

Lunch: Quinoa salad with chickpeas, diced vegetables, and a lemon-tahini dressing.

Evening Bite: Cut cucumber with curds.

Dinner: Barbecued shrimp or heated cod with steamed vegetables.

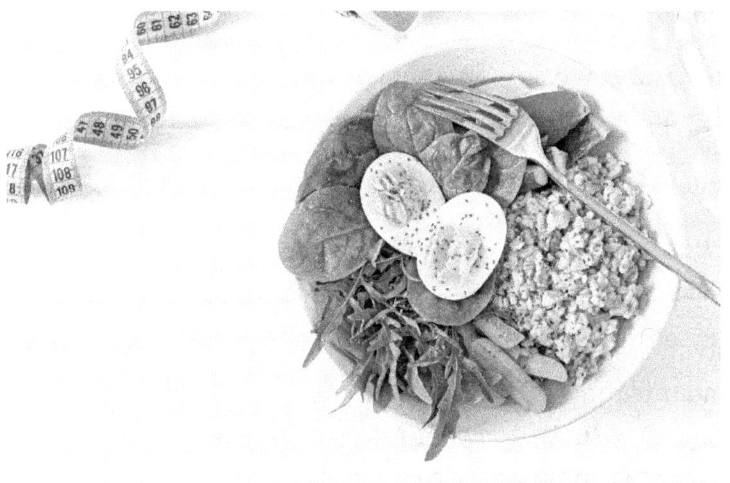

Week 3:

Breakfast: Smoothie with spinach, banana, almond milk, and a scoop of protein powder.

Early in the day bite: A little bowl of blended berries.

Lunch: Lentil soup with a side of blended green serving of mixed greens.

Evening Tidbit: Greek yogurt with a shower of honey and a couple of cuts of kiwi.

Dinner: Prepared chicken or tofu with yams and broccoli.

Week 4:

Breakfast: Short-term oats with chia seeds, almond milk, and a new organic product.

Early in the day bite: A modest bunch of pumpkin seeds or sunflower seeds.

Lunch: Earthy-colored rice bowl with dark beans, avocado, salsa, and a sprinkle of cheddar.

Evening Bite: Cut ringer peppers with guacamole.

Dinner: Barbecued steak or Portobello mushrooms with broiled Brussels sprouts.

Notwithstanding the eating regimen graph, make sure to remain hydrated by drinking a lot of water over the day. Lessen or dispose of sweet refreshments and select natural teas or implanted water all things being equal.

Kindly recollect that this diet graph is not a substitute for proficient clinical guidance. It means quite a bit to work with a medical services supplier or an enrolled dietitian to make a customized plan that tends to your particular well-being needs and objectives. They can likewise screen your headway and make changes on a case-by-case basis during the 30-day challenge.

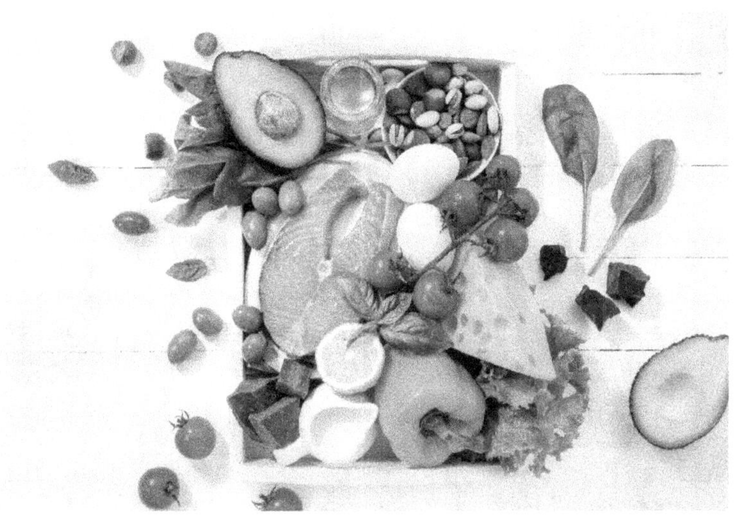

HOW I DO GET MY IRREGULAR PERIODS BACK TO NORMAL?

I comprehend that managing unpredictable periods can be disturbing, and you might be looking for ways of restoring your feminine cycle once again. Here are a few general advances you can take, yet if it's not too much trouble, make sure to counsel a medical care supplier for customized exhortation and to preclude any fundamental ailments:

Counsel a Medical Services Supplier: The first and most urgent step is to see a gynecologist or medical care supplier. They can assist with distinguishing the fundamental reason for your sporadic periods and foster a treatment plan given your particular requirements.

Hormonal Contraception: Contingent upon the reason for your unpredictable periods, your medical services supplier might prescribe hormonal contraception to direct your feminine cycle.

Way of life Changes: Certain way of life changes can decidedly affect feminine routineness. Center around keeping a reasonable eating routine, taking part in ordinary activity, overseeing pressure, and getting satisfactory rest.

Keep a Solid Weight: On the off chance that you are underweight or overweight, accomplishing a solid weight might assist with controlling your periods.

Oversee Pressure: Ongoing pressure can disturb the hormonal equilibrium and feminine cycles. Practice pressure-decreasing strategies like contemplation, yoga, profound breathing activities, or side interests you appreciate.

Address Fundamental Medical Issue: Conditions like polycystic ovary disorder (PCOS), thyroid issues, or other hormonal awkward nature can cause unpredictable periods. Treating these circumstances can assist with normalizing your feminine cycle.

Drug Survey: A few drugs can influence feminine consistency. On the off chance that you are taking any prescriptions, talk about them with your medical services supplier to check whether changes are vital.

Homegrown Enhancements: A few homegrown supplements, such as chaste berry (Vitex), have been generally used to help chemical equilibrium. Nonetheless, consistently talk with your medical care supplier before attempting any enhancements.

WHAT IS THE BEST TREATMENT FOR IRREGULAR PERIODS?

The best treatment for sporadic periods relies upon the basic reason. It is fundamental to counsel a medical care supplier to decide the particular reason and get customized therapy, which might incorporate hormonal conception prevention, way of life changes, drug, or tending to hidden ailments.

The Menstrual Cycle

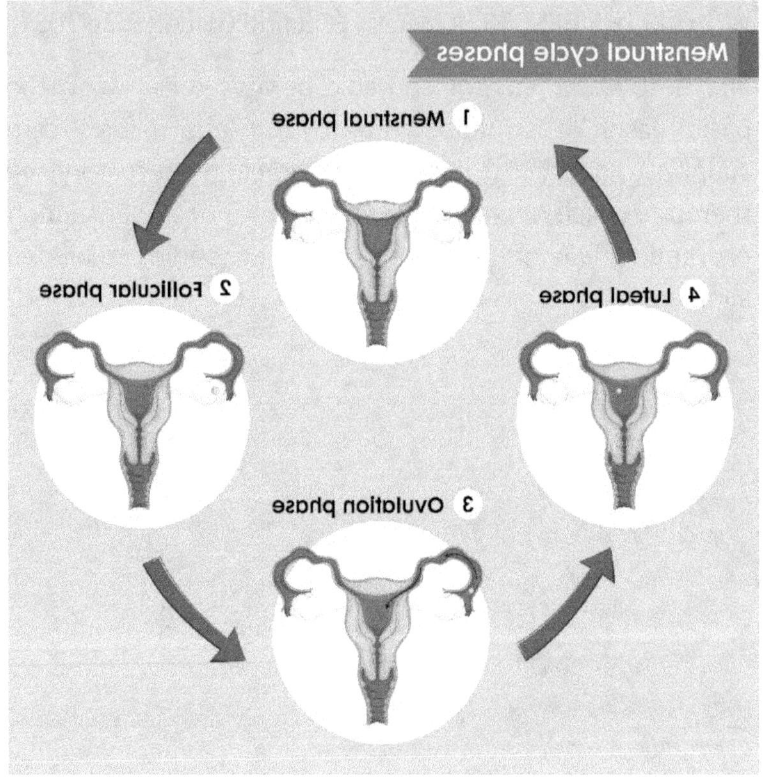

The feminine cycle is a complex physiological cycle that happens in fruitful people with female conceptive frameworks. It assumes a pivotal part in human multiplication and ripeness. Since forever ago, the feminine cycle has been dependent upon different social and cultural insights, prompting the two misconceptions and strengthening them. This far-reaching part means giving a top-to-bottom examination of the monthly cycle, covering its definition, stages, hormonal guideline, related side effects, feminine issues, and the effect of social perspectives and medical care. By understanding this central part of female physiology, we can scatter misinterpretations, advance conceptive well-being, and cultivate a more comprehensive and informed society.

Introduction:

The monthly cycle is a characteristic peculiarity remarkable to people with female conceptive frameworks. It includes a progression of occasions happening roughly like clockwork, however, varieties in cycle length are normal. The cycle is set apart by variances in chemicals and changes in the regenerative organs, setting up the body for expected pregnancy. It is fundamental to investigate the feminine cycle from various points to see the value of its importance in human well-being and propagation. The monthly cycle is a characteristic interaction that happens in ladies of regenerative age. An intricate cycle is constrained by chemicals, and it ordinarily goes on for 28 days. The period has four stages: period, the follicular stage, ovulation, and the luteal stage

- **MENSTRAL PHASE**

  The feminine stage is the principal phase of the period and imprints the start of the cycle. It is likewise usually known as the monthly cycle or the period. During this stage, the body sheds the inward covering of the uterus, called the endometrium, which has developed in anticipation of a possible pregnancy in the past cycle. If pregnancy doesn't happen, the body removes this coating through the vagina as feminine blood.

Duration:

The feminine stage ordinarily goes on for around 3 to 7 days, albeit individual varieties can happen. The typical length of a monthly cycle is something like 5 days.

Hormonal Changes:

Toward the start of the feminine stage, chemical levels, especially estrogen, and progesterone, are at their most minimal. This decrease in chemical levels sets off the shedding of the endometrial coating.

Feminine Blood:

The feminine blood comprises blood, tissue from the uterine coating, and cervical bodily fluid. The shade of feminine blood can fluctuate from dazzling red to dim brown, with the stream being heavier during the initial not many days and continuously diminishing as the stage advances.

Feminine Side Effects:

During this stage, a few people might encounter different physical and close-to-home side effects, all in all, known as premenstrual condition (PMS). Normal side effects incorporate stomach cramps, bosom delicacy, bulging, migraines, weakness, peevishness, and emotional episodes.

Feminine Cleanliness:

Keeping up with legitimate feminine cleanliness is pivotal during this stage to forestall contaminations and uneasiness. Utilizing sterile cushions, tampons, feminine cups, or period undies is fundamental to ingesting feminine blood and keeping up with neatness. Cleanliness practices, for example, changing feminine items routinely and it is mean a lot to wash the genital region.

Ripeness and Pregnancy:

The feminine stage is viewed as a low-richness period since ovulation has not yet happened. Notwithstanding, it is as yet workable for pregnancy to result from sex during this stage, as sperm can make due in the regenerative plot for a few days

- **FOLLICULAR PHASE**

The follicular stage is the primary period of the feminine cycle. It starts on the primary day of your period and closes with ovulation. During the follicular stage, an egg develops in one of your ovaries. The egg is contained in a little sac called a follicle. The follicle delivers the chemical estrogen, which makes the coating of your uterus thicken in anticipation of a potential pregnancy.

The follicular stage regularly goes on for 14 days, yet it can change from one lady to another. The length of the follicular stage is impacted by various elements, including age, body weight, and feelings of anxiety.

Side effects of the follicular stage

A few ladies experience gentle side effects during the follicular stage, for example,
Expanded vaginal release
Bosom delicacy
Cramps
Clear or smooth vaginal release
Expanded sex drive
These side effects are generally gentle and disappear all alone. Be that as it may, on the off chance that you experience any extreme side effects, for example, weighty draining or serious torment, you ought to converse with your primary care physician.

Chemicals during the follicular stage

The fundamental chemicals that are associated with the follicular stage are estrogen and follicle-animating chemicals (FSH). FSH is delivered by the pituitary organ in the mind. It animates the development of follicles in the ovaries. As the follicles mature, they produce expanding levels of estrogen. Estrogen makes the covering of the uterus thicken in anticipation of a potential pregnancy.

- **OVULATION PHASE**
  Ovulation is the third phase of the menstrual cycle. It is the time when a mature egg is   released from one of the ovaries. Ovulation typically occurs 14 days before the start of the next menstrual period.

However, the timing of ovulation can vary from woman to woman.

Ovulation symptoms

Some women experience mild symptoms during ovulation, such as:

- Cervical mucus: The cervical mucus becomes clear and stretchy during ovulation, which can make it easier for sperm to travel through the cervix and into the uterus.
- Basal body temperature: The basal body temperature (BBT) may rise slightly after ovulation.
- Ovulation pain: Some women experience mild pain in the lower abdomen or pelvis during ovulation.

Hormones during ovulation

The main hormones that are involved in ovulation are luteinizing hormone (LH) and follicle-stimulating hormone (FSH). FSH stimulates the growth of follicles in the ovaries. As the follicles mature, they produce increasing levels of estrogen. Estrogen causes the lining of the uterus to thicken in preparation for a possible pregnancy.

LH levels surge just before ovulation. This surge of LH triggers the release of the egg from the ovary. The egg then travels through the fallopian tube towards the uterus.

Implantation

If the egg is fertilized by a sperm, it will implant in the lining of the uterus about 6-12 days after ovulation. The fertilized egg will then begin to produce the hormone human chorionic gonadotropin (HCG). HCG helps to maintain the corpus Lu-teum, which continues to produce progesterone. Progesterone helps to support the pregnancy until the placenta is formed.

If the egg is not fertilized, the corpus Lu-teum will break down and the levels of progesterone will fall. This will cause the lining of the uterus to shed and menstruation will begin again.

If you are trying to conceive, it is important to track your ovulation. This will help you to identify the days when you are most likely to be fertile. There are several ways to track your ovulation, including:

- Keeping a menstrual calendar: This is a simple way to track the start and end dates of your menstrual periods.
- Using a menstrual app: There are several menstrual apps available that can help you to track your cycle. These apps typically allow you to track your period, your ovulation, and your symptoms.
- Taking ovulation predictor kits (OPKs): OPKs are test strips that measure the levels of LH in your urine. LH levels surge just before ovulation, so using an OPK can help you to identify the day of ovulation.

- **LUTERAL Stage**

  The luteal stage is the fourth and last period of the monthly cycle. It starts after ovulation and closures with the beginning of your next feminine period. During the luteal stage, the corpus Lu-teum,a little organ that structures in the ovary after ovulation, creates the chemical progesterone. Progesterone assists with keeping up with the coating of your uterus in anticipation of a potential pregnancy. On the off chance that the egg isn't prepared, the corpus Lu-teum will separate and the degrees of progesterone will fall. This will make the covering of the uterus shed and monthly cycle will start in the future.

The luteal stage regularly goes on for 14 days, however it can shift from one lady to another. The length of the luteal stage is impacted by various variables, including age, body weight, and feelings of anxiety.

Side effects of the luteal stage
A few ladies experience gentle side effects during the luteal stage, for example,
Bosom delicacy
Cramps
Weakness
Food desires
Mind-set swings
These side effects are generally gentle and disappear all alone. Be that as it may, on the off chance that you experience any extreme side effects, for example, weighty draining or serious torment, you ought to converse with your primary care physician.

Chemicals during the luteal stage
The primary chemicals that are associated with the luteal stage are progesterone and luteinizing chemical (LH). LH is delivered by the pituitary organ in the cerebrum. It animates the arrival of the egg from the ovary during ovulation. After ovulation, the corpus Lu-teum produces progesterone. Progesterone assists with keeping up with the covering of the uterus in anticipation of a potential pregnancy.

Implantation

Assuming the egg is prepared, it will embed in the covering of the uterus around 6-12 days after ovulation. The prepared egg will then start to deliver the chemical human chorionic gonadotropin (HCG). HCG assists with keeping up with the corpus Lu-teum, which keeps on delivering progesterone. Progesterone assists with supporting the pregnancy until the placenta is shaped.

On the off chance that the egg isn't prepared

On the off chance that the egg isn't prepared, the corpus Lu-teum will separate and the degrees of progesterone will fall. This will make the covering of the uterus shed and monthly cycle will start in the future.

Following your luteal stage

In the event that you are attempting to consider, following your luteal phase is significant. This will assist you with recognizing the days when you are probably going to be rich. There are various ways of following your luteal stage, including:

Keeping a feminine schedule: This is a straightforward method for following the beginning and end dates of your feminine periods.

Utilizing a feminine application: There are various feminine applications accessible that can assist you with following your cycle. These applications commonly permit you to follow your period, your ovulation, and your side effects.

Taking ovulation indicator units (OPKs): OPKs are test strips that action the degrees of LH in your pee. LH levels flood not long before ovulation, so utilizing an OPK can assist you with distinguishing the day of ovulation.

PART 2
5 Yoga Poses for a Healthy Menstrual Cycle

Yoga is a mind-body exercise that has numerous health benefits for women. Strengthening, increasing flexibility, and lowering stress are all benefits. Additionally, yoga can help with menstrual symptoms like cramping, bloating, and exhaustion.

There are several yoga postures that can support a regular periods improved our cycle.

1 Cat-Cow Pose:

Feline cow present is a delicate yoga representation that is an extraordinary method for extending the spine and further developing adaptability. It is likewise an effective method for easing pressure and strain.

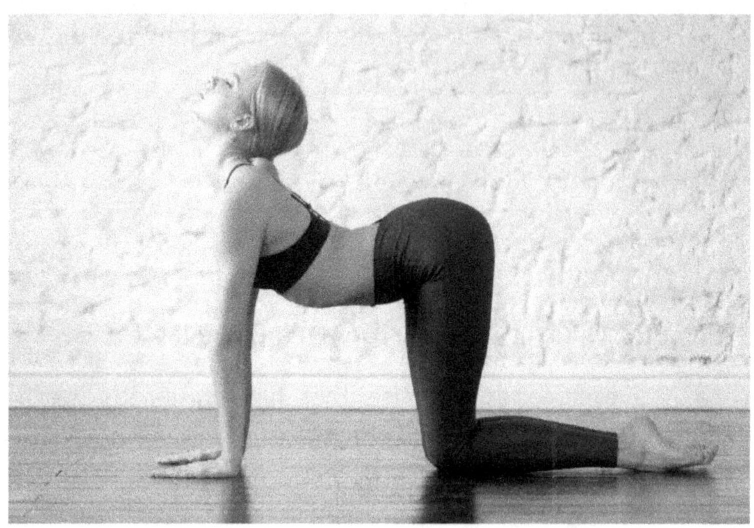

To do a feline cow present, begin on your hands and knees. Your hands ought to be shoulder-width separated and your knees ought to be hip-width separated. Breathe in and curve your back like a feline, getting your jaw into your chest. Breathe out and adjust your back like a cow, dropping your head down and looking between your knees. Rehash this development a few times, taking in as you curve your back and out as you round your back.

Advantages of feline cow present:

Further develops adaptability in the spine

Assuages pressure and strain

Assists with opening up the chest

Fortifies the center

Further develops act

Step-by-step instructions to do feline cow present:

Begin your hands and knees, with your hands shoulder-width separated and your knees hip-width

separated.

Breathe in and curve your back, getting your jawline into your chest.

Breathe out and adjust your back, dropping your head down and looking between your knees.

Rehash this development a few times, taking in as you curve your back and out as you round your back.

Hold each posture for a couple of breaths.

Precautions:

Assuming you have any back aggravation, begin this posture gradually and try not to curve your back something over the top.

Assuming you have any neck torment, try not to drop your head down something over the top.

Assuming you are pregnant, keep away from this posture in the principal trimester.

Modifications:

Assuming you are new to yoga, you can begin by essentially adjusting and angling your back without lifting your head.

Assuming you experience issues adjusting on all fours, you can do this posture from your knees.

If you have any wrist torment, you can put your hands on blocks or a yoga mat.

Variations:

You can add wind to the feline cow present by contorting your middle to the right as you curve your back and to the left as you round your back.

You can likewise add a pelvic slant to the feline cow present by tucking your pelvis under as you curve your back and delivering your pelvis as you round your back.

2 Pigeon Pose:

Pigeon Posture, otherwise called Eka Pada Rajakapotasana in Sanskrit, is a famous yoga representation that gives a profound stretch to the hips and thighs. It is named after the likeness of the situation to a pigeon's stance. This yoga present is ordinarily rehearsed in different styles of yoga, including Hatha, Vinyasa, and Ashtanga. Pigeon Posture offers various physical and mental advantages and is many times remembered for yoga arrangements to upgrade adaptability, discharge strain, and advance unwinding.

Here is a bit-by-bit guide on the most proficient method to rehearse Pigeon Posture:

Beginning Position:

Start in a tabletop position with your hands and knees on the mat. Adjust your wrists under your shoulders and your knees under your hips. Guarantee that your spine is in an unbiased position.

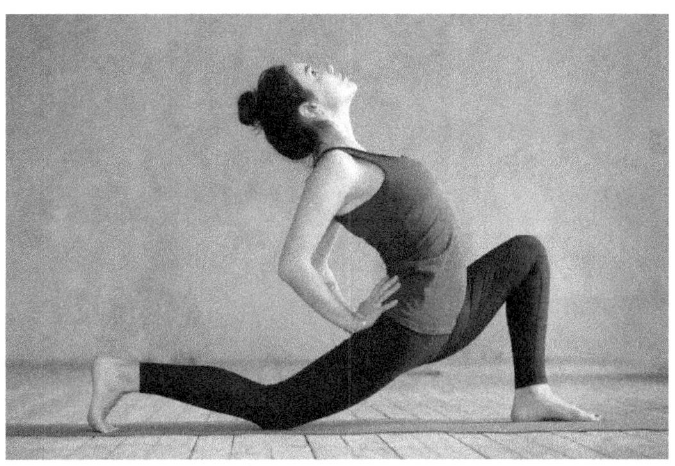

Progress to Pigeon Posture:

Present your right knee and spot it behind your right wrist. The right foot ought to be calculated somewhat slantingly and by the left hip. The shin of your right leg ought to be on the mat, and the foot ought to be flexed.

Leg Arrangement:

Slide your left leg straight back, bringing down the front of your passed-on thigh to the mat. The highest point of your left foot ought to lie on the floor.

Hip Arrangement:

Make sure that your right hip is remotely pivoted, and the left hip is inside turned. Mean to have the two hips squared to the front of the mat. This arrangement safeguards the knee joint and considers a more profound stretch.

Extend the Spine:

Breathe in profoundly and lengthen your spine, lifting your chest and expanding your sternum forward. Connect with your center to help your lower back.

Forward Overlap:

As you breathe out, start to walk your hands forward, gradually bringing down your middle over your right leg. Keep your hips square and try not to fall on the right side.

Resting Position:

When you track down an agreeable edge, lay your brow on the mat or utilize a block or pad for help. You can likewise put your lower arms on the mat for a more profound stretch.

Breathing and Unwinding:

Remain in the posture for 5 to 10 breaths, permitting your body to unwind and deliver strain. Center around profound and consistent breathing, relinquishing any physical or mental strain.

Switch Sides:

To emerge from the posture, draw in your center and walk your hands back, lifting your chest area. Then, fold your back toes, and step your right foot back to the tabletop position. Rehash a similar grouping on the opposite side, presenting your left knee.

Alterations and Varieties:

If you find it trying to overlay forward totally, utilize a prop, for example, a block or pad to help your chest area.

For a more extraordinary stretch, you can attempt the Lord Pigeon Posture (Kapotasana), which includes arriving at the back to hold your back foot with two hands.

Advantages of Pigeon Posture:

Extends the hip flexors, thighs, and crotches.

Opens the hips and increments hip adaptability.

Lightens strain in the lower back and hips.

Animates stomach organs and further develop assimilation.

Discharges profound and mental pressure put away in the hips.

Readies the body for situated contemplation.

Precautions:

Try not to rehearse Pigeon Posture if you have a new knee or hip injury.

Assuming you feel any aggravation or distress in your knees, use props or alter the posture to suit your body's necessities.

Continuously pay attention to your body and try not to drive yourself into the posture over your agreeable brink.

Similarly, as with any yoga representation, it's crucial for training Pigeon Posture carefully and with consciousness of your body's limits. Integrate this hip-opening posture into your yoga routine to encounter its various advantages for both the body and psyche.

3 Spinal Twist Pose:

Spinal wind present (otherwise called ardha matsyendrasana) is a yoga representation that is an incredible method for extending the spine and further developing adaptability. It is likewise an effective method for easing pressure and strain.

To do spinal wind present, begin sitting on the floor with your legs stretched out before you. Twist your right knee and carry your right foot to the beyond your left thigh. Put your right hand behind you on the floor for help. Shelter the right, bringing your left arm over your right thigh and your abandoned hand to the ground. You can likewise put your left hand on your right knee for help. Hold the posture for a couple of breaths, then recurrent on the opposite side.

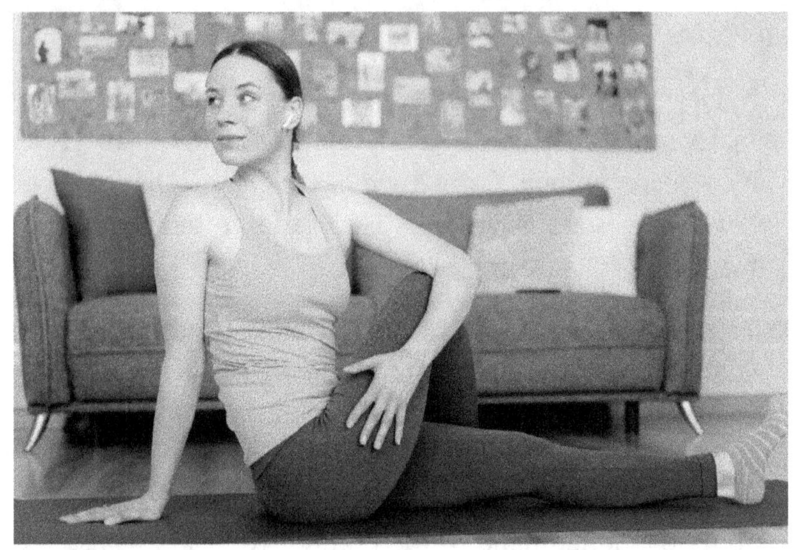

Advantages of spinal contort present:

Further develops adaptability in the spine

Alleviates pressure and strain

Assists with opening up the ches

Sit on the floor with your legs stretched out before you.

Twist your right knee and carry your right foot to the beyond your left thigh.

Put your right hand behind you on the floor for help.

Shelter the right, bringing your left arm over your right thigh and your abandoned hand to the ground.

Hold the posture for a couple of breaths, then, at that point, rehash on the opposite side.

Precautions:

On the off chance that you have any back aggravation, begin this posture gradually and abstain from curving excessively.

On the off chance that you have any neck torment, try not to drop your head excessively.

Assuming you are pregnant, keep away from this posture in the principal trimester.

Modifications:

Assuming that you are new to yoga, you can begin by essentially winding your middle to one side without lifting your arm.

If you experience issues adjusting your sit bones, you can sit on a block or a cushion.

If you have any wrist torment, you can put your hands kneeling down or on blocks.

Variations:

You can add a curve to the spinal bend present by winding your middle to the right as you breathe in and to the left as you breathe out.

You can likewise add a pelvic slant to the spinal contort present by tucking your pelvis under as you curve to the right and delivering your pelvis as you wind to the left.

- **CORPSE POSE**

  Carcass present (otherwise called shavasana) is a yoga representation that is an incredible method for unwinding and de-stress. It is an inactive posture, implying that you don't have to successfully keep up with it.

  To do a cadaver present, begin by lying on your back with your legs broadened and your arms at your sides. Shut your eyes and loosen up your whole body. You can inhale profoundly and gradually, or you can essentially notice your breath. Hold the posture however long you like.

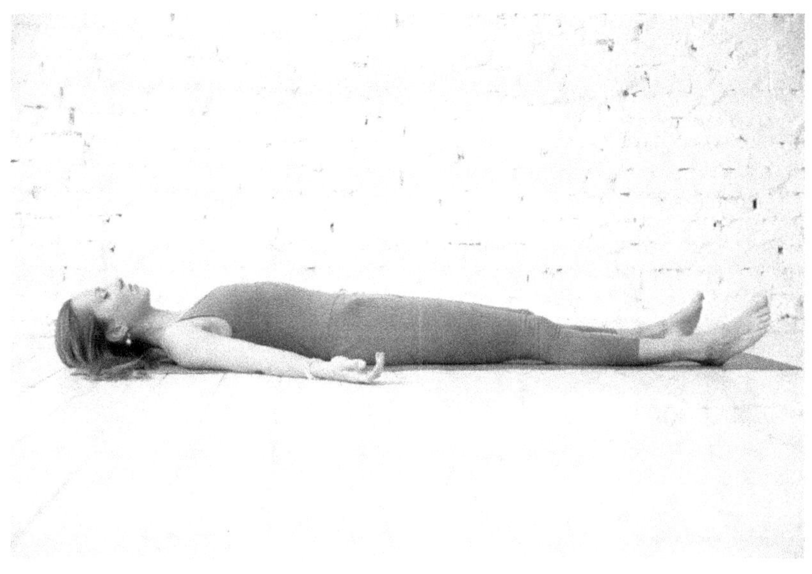

Advantages of corpse present:

Loosens up the body and psyche

Lessens pressure and uneasiness

Further develops rest

Further develops dissemination

Discharges muscle pressure

The most effective method to do cadaver present:

Lie on your back with your legs expanded and your arms at your sides.

Shut your eyes and loosen up your whole body.

Inhale profoundly and gradually, or just notice your breath.

Hold the posture however long you like.

Precautions:

If you have any neck torment, you can put a rolled-up towel under your neck.

Assuming that you have any lower back torment, you can twist your knees and put your feet level on the floor.

On the off chance that you are pregnant, you can put a cushion under your knees.

Modifications:

On the off chance that you are new to yoga, you can begin by just lying on your back and shutting your eyes.

If you experience issues unwinding, you can take a stab at counting your breaths or zeroing in on your breath.

Assuming you have any aggravation, you can change your situation or alter your posture.

Variations:

You can add a contort to the carcass present by putting your right hand on your left side hip and your left hand on your right hip. Delicately curve your middle to the right, then to the left.

You can likewise add a pelvic slant to the cadaver present by tucking your pelvis under as you breathe in and delivering your pelvis as you breathe out.

3 Yoga Nidra:

Yoga Nidra, often referred to as "yogic sleep," is a powerful relaxation and meditation technique that originates from the ancient yogic tradition. It is a state of conscious deep relaxation, where the practitioner hovers between wakefulness and sleep, inducing a profound state of calmness and awareness. The practice of Yoga Nidra allows the mind and body to enter a state of profound relaxation, promoting healing, restoration, and self-discovery.

Yoga Nidra is typically guided by a facilitator or instructor who provides verbal instructions throughout the practice. The practitioner lies down in a comfortable position, such as Savasana (corpse pose), with eyes closed, and listens to the instructor's guidance. The practice can last anywhere from 20 minutes to an hour or more, depending on the session's purpose and the practitioner's experience.

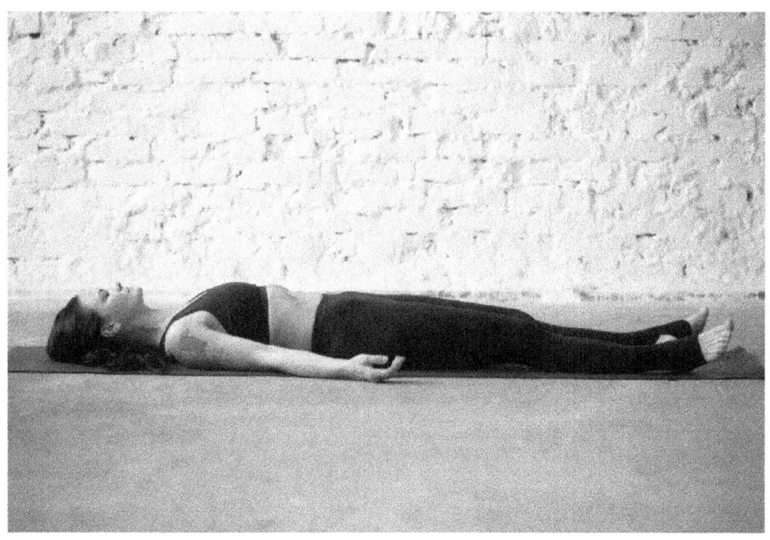

Key Elements of Yoga Nidra:

1. Intention Setting: The practice often begins with the practitioner setting an intention or Sankalpa for the session. This intention acts as a positive affirmation or a personal goal, and it is mentally repeated at the beginning and end of the practice to reinforce its effects on the subconscious mind.
2. Rotation of Awareness: During the practice, the instructor guides the practitioner's awareness through different parts of the body systematically. The practitioner brings their attention to each body part, experiencing sensations without any judgment or effort to change them.
3. Breath Awareness: Conscious breathing is an integral part of Yoga Nidra. Practitioners are encouraged to observe their breath and allow it to become slow, deep, and rhythmic, which further enhances relaxation and reduces stress.
4. Visualization: The practice may incorporate guided imagery to stimulate the mind's creative and intuitive faculties. Visualization techniques help to access the subconscious mind and unlock inner potential.
5. Intention Manifestation: Towards the end of the practice, the practitioner revisits their initial intention or Sankalpa. This repetition during the deeply relaxed state helps to plant the seed of positive change in the subconscious mind.

Benefits of Yoga Nidra:

1. Stress Reduction: Yoga Nidra activates the parasympathetic nervous system, triggering the

relaxation response and reducing stress and anxiety.

2. Improved Sleep: Regular practice of Yoga Nidra can improve the quality of sleep and help with insomnia and sleep-related issues.
3. Enhanced Concentration and Memory: The practice helps to improve focus, concentration, and memory by calming the mind and reducing mental chatter.
4. Emotional Healing: Yoga Nidra allows practitioners to explore and release suppressed emotions, promoting emotional healing and well-being.
5. Increased Self-Awareness: The practice encourages self-reflection and introspection, leading to a deeper understanding of oneself.

Yoga Nidra is accessible to individuals of all ages and fitness levels. It is especially beneficial for those experiencing high levels of stress, and anxiety, or seeking deep relaxation and inner exploration. Since it requires only a comfortable space and the ability to listen, it can be practiced at home, in yoga studios, or even at the workplace during breaks.

PART 3

BREATHING Techniques for a Healthy Menstrual Cycle

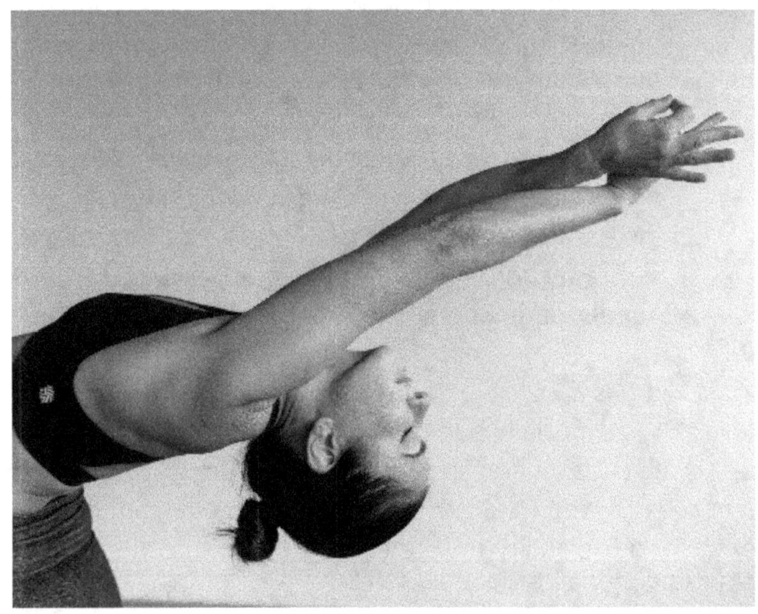

A sound monthly cycle is fundamental for a lady's general prosperity, as it impacts her physical, close-to-home, and psychological wellness. Hormonal vacillations during the period can prompt different side effects, like issues, bulging, state of mind swings, and weakness. Be that as it may, rehearsing explicit breathing procedures can fundamentally add to a smoother and better feminine experience. This far-reaching guide investigates the significance of breathing methods in keeping a fair feminine cycle and gives itemized directions on the most proficient method to carry out them.

Area 1: Figuring out the Period

Before diving into the breathing methods, understanding the periods of the feminine cycle is vital:

Feminine Stage: This stage includes the shedding of the uterine coating and ordinarily goes on for 3-7 days.

Follicular Stage: During this stage, the body gets ready for ovulation, and the follicles in the ovaries mature.

Ovulatory Stage: Ovulation happens during this short stage when a full-grown egg is set free from the ovary.

Luteal Stage: On the off chance that the egg isn't treated, the body enters the luteal stage, where the uterine covering thickens to help an expected pregnancy.

Segment 2: The Association between Breathing and the Period

Breathing methods significantly affect the autonomic sensory system, which directs fundamental physical processes not under cognizant control. The two essential parts of the autonomic sensory system are the thoughtful (survival) and parasympathetic (rest and review) frameworks. Stress and nervousness actuate the thoughtful framework while unwinding and smoothness enact the parasympathetic framework.

Persistent pressure can upset the hormonal equilibrium in the body, influencing the feminine cycle. By integrating explicit breathing strategies, ladies can animate the parasympathetic sensory system, diminishing pressure and advancing hormonal equilibrium during each feminine stage.

Segment 3: Breathing Methods for a Sound Feminine Cycle

Profound Stomach Breathing (Diaphragmatic Relaxing):

Sit or rests serenely, putting one hand on your chest and the other on your paunch.

Breathe in profoundly through your nose, permitting your paunch to rise and grow, while your chest remains generally still.

Breathe out leisurely through your mouth, feeling your midsection fall internally.

Practice this for 5-10 minutes day to day, particularly during the feminine stage, to decrease squeezes and advance unwinding.

Substitute Nostril Breathing (Nadi Shodhana):

Sit in an agreeable position and utilize your right thumb to close your right nostril.

Breathe in profoundly through your left nostril.

Close your left nostril with your right ring finger, delivering the right nostril.

Breathe out through your right nostril.

Breathe in through your right nostril.

Close your right nostril, delivering the left nostril.

Breathe out through your left nostril.

This method adjusts the left and right sides of the equator of the mind and directs hormonal vacillations.

Ujjayi Breath (Sea Breath):

Sit or remain with a casual stance.

Breathe in profoundly through your nose, marginally tightening the rear of your throat, making a delicate sea-like sound.

Breathe out leisurely through your nose, keeping up with the choking in your throat.

Ujjayi breath quiets the psyche and decreases nervousness, which can be helpful during the ovulatory and luteal stages.

Honey bee Breath (Bhramari Pranayama):

Track down an agreeable situated position and shut your eyes.

Place your fingers tenderly over your eyes, your pointers laying on your eyebrows.

Breathe in profoundly through your nose.

Breathe out leisurely while making a murmuring sound like a honey bee, permitting the vibration to calm your brain.

This breath work is magnificent for lightening emotional episodes and nervousness during the period.

Cooling Breath (Shitali Pranayama):

Sit easily, broadening your tongue outside your mouth, twisting the edges to frame a cylinder.

Breathe in profoundly through the cylinder-like tongue.

Hold your breath momentarily.

Close your mouth and breathe out leisurely through your nose.

Shitali Pranayama helps cool the body, lessening crabbiness and intensity-related distress during the feminine stage.

Area 4: The Significance of Consistency

Consistency is key while working on breathing methods for a solid monthly cycle. The day-to-day practice of these methods, particularly during the feminine stage, can yield long-haul benefits. By incorporating these practices into your day-to-day daily schedule, you can make a positive effect on your hormonal equilibrium, profound prosperity, and actual well-being.

Breathing methods are incredible assets that can essentially impact a lady's feminine cycle and general well-being. By embracing these practices with devotion and consistency, ladies can encounter diminished feminine distress, better close-to-home guideline, and a superior feeling of prosperity. Similarly, as with any new practice, it's fundamental to counsel medical services proficiently before starting, particularly if you have any basic medical issue. In this way, take a full breath, embrace these strategies, and engage yourself to have a better monthly cycle and a more joyful life.

PART 4

Meditation for a Healthy Menstrual Cycle

Contemplation or meditation can be a useful practice to help a sound monthly cycle by decreasing pressure, advancing unwinding, and improving by and large prosperity. Stress and tension can adversely influence chemical levels and a feminine consistency, so integrating contemplation into your routine might assist with establishing a more adjusted hormonal climate. You can try the following meditation techniques:

Care Contemplation: Care contemplation includes carrying your complete focus to the current second without judgment. Sit comfortably in a quiet location and concentrate on your breath. If your psyche begins to meander, delicately take your consideration back to your breath. Ordinary practice can assist with diminishing pressure and advance profound steadiness.

Directed Perception: This includes envisioning yourself in a quiet climate. Imagine a calm beach or beautiful forest where you feel safe and at ease. Keep your eyes closed. Connect every one of your faculties in the representation to make it more clear and vivid.

Body Output Reflection: Sit comfortably or lie down, and gradually pay attention to various parts of your body. Begin from your toes and move gradually up to your head, seeing any pressure or inconvenience. Allow those areas to relax and let go of any tension by breathing into them.

Adoring Benevolence Reflection: This training includes developing sensations of affection and sympathy towards yourself as well as other people. While contemplating, rehash positive attestations or expressions like, "May I be sound and blissful," "May my body track down equilibrium and agreement," or whatever other assertions that impact you.

Chakra Contemplation: This sort of reflection centers around the energy communities in your body known as chakras. Different aspects of physical and emotional health are linked to each chakra. Concentrating on these energy points can aid in healing and balance. You can find directed chakra contemplation meetings on the web.

Practices in Breathing: Breathing deeply and slowly can help ease stress and calm the nervous system. Breathe deeply into your belly using your nose to fill your diaphragm and slowly exhale through your mouth to practice deep belly breathing. Count your breaths to keep up with the center.

Yoga Nidra: Otherwise called yogic rest, this training includes resting in an agreeable position and following a directed contemplation that takes you through various phases of unwinding. It can assist in stress reduction and deep relaxation.

Notwithstanding these particular sorts of contemplation, there are likewise some broad reflection rehearses that can be useful for feminine well-being. These include:

Performing frequently: The more you reflect, the more advantages you will probably insight. Intend to ponder for something like 10 minutes out of each day, however, longer meetings can be significantly more valuable.

Tracking down an agreeable position: Sitting or lying in a position that allows you to concentrate on your meditation practice should be possible.

Learning to meditate effectively takes time: Try not to get deterred on the off chance that you don't get results right away. Simply continue to practice and you will ultimately begin to receive the rewards.

Reflection is a protected and successful method for overseeing feminine side effects and advancing generally feminine well-being. If you are searching for a characteristic method for working on your feminine cycle, reflection is an extraordinary choice to consider.

Here are a few extra ways to involve reflection for feminine well-being:

Select a time of day when you are most likely to focus and relax.

Find a calm spot where you won't be upset.

Wear happy with apparel that won't confine your development.

Assuming you are new to contemplation, begin with short meetings and slowly increment the length of your training over the long haul.

Be patient and predictable with your training.

Here is a portion of the advantages of contemplation for feminine well-being:

Easy menstrual discomfort: Reflection can assist with decreasing the force of feminine spasms and other torment related to the monthly cycle.

Further develops state of mind: Menstrual symptoms can both benefit from mood enhancement and stress reduction through meditation.

Aid in relaxation: Reflection can assist with advancing unwinding and decreasing pressure, which can be useful for diminishing feminine side effects.

Further develops rest: Meditation can help alleviate menstrual symptoms and improve the quality of sleep.

Increments mindfulness: Contemplation can assist with expanding mindfulness, which can be useful for understanding and overseeing feminine side effects.

FINAL PART

Tips for Practicing Yoga for Menstrual Health

Yoga is a great way to improve your overall health and well-being, and it can also be beneficial for menstrual health. Here are some tips and tricks for practicing yoga for menstrual health. Here are a few hints and deceives for rehearsing yoga for feminine well-being.

Begin slowly: If you are new to yoga, begin with delicate postures and bit by bit increment the force as you become more agreeable.

Pay attention to your body: Assuming you are feeling torment, stop the posture and rest. There is a compelling reason need to propel yourself excessively hard.

Select supportive postures: A few postures, for example, feline cow and youngster's posture, can be particularly useful for easing feminine spasms.

Take note of your breath: Yoga can assist you with unwinding and center around your breath, which can be useful for diminishing pressure and working on generally speaking feminine well-being.

Show restraint: The benefits of yoga for menstrual health take time to become apparent. Be patient and reliable with your training, and you will ultimately begin to get results.

The following are a few particular poses that can be beneficial to menstrual health:

Feline cow present: Stretching the spine and releasing tension are both aided by this pose.

The child poses: This posture is an incredible method for unwinding and discharging pressure.

Pigeon present: Menstrual cramps can be alleviated and hips can be opened with this pose.

Bridge position: Improved circulation and core strength are two benefits of this pose.

Savasana: This posture is an extraordinary method for unwinding and de-stress. Use Props: Yoga props like blocks, reinforces, and covers can be useful in offering help and making your training more open during your period.

Concentrate on Your Breath and Meditate: Integrate pranayama (breath work) and contemplation into your training. Profound breathing and reflection can assist with quieting the sensory system and lessen pressure, which can be especially advantageous during periods.

Remain Hydrated: Drink a lot of water previously, during, and after your training to remain hydrated, particularly during your feminine period.

Rest when Required: It is acceptable to take a day off or engage in gentle yoga or meditation rather than a more strenuous routine if you are feeling exhausted or lacking in energy.

Keep in mind that every woman has a different experience with her menstrual cycle, so it's important to figure out what works best for you. On the off chance that you have particular clinical worries or conditions connected with your feminine well-being, it's dependably smart to talk with medical services proficient before beginning or changing your yoga practice.

On the off chance that you are new to yoga, it is smart, to begin with a novice yoga class or to work with a certified yoga educator. They can assist you with picking represents that are appropriate for you and adjust acts as required.